T5-CQD-197

{Hope and Destiny Jr.}

The Adolescent's Guide to Sickle Cell Diseases

{Abridged Booklet Edition}

Lewis L. Hsu, MD, PhD

Silvia R. Brandalise, MD

Carmen C. M. Rodrigues, RN

Hilton Publishing · Chicago, IL

Contents

What is Sickle Cell Disease?

How do kids get SCD?

More than 70,000 Americans have sickle cell disease today, and about 90% of those cases are in people of African descent. Unpredictable and sometimes severe pain attacks are the most common symptom experienced by people with sickle cell disease and, at times, the pain may require hospitalization so strong medications may be administered to the patient. Other health issues related to sickle cell disease include strokes, lung damage, severe anemia and serious infections.

There are several types of sickle cell disease

In the most common type of sickle cell disease in the United States and most countries, the gene for sickle hemoglobin is inherited from both parents and results in the production of only abnormal sickle hemoglobin. This is called sickle cell disease, SS type. It is also called sickle cell anemia.

The same sickling of red blood cells shows up in lesser-known forms of the disease as well. The SC type, often called "SC disease," and sickle beta thalassemia, or "S beta thal" or "sickle beta thal," are quite common. In sickle cell disease SC, one parent passes down the gene for sickle hemoglobin, while the other parent contributes the gene for the abnormal C type of hemoglobin.

Similarly, a child with S beta thal also has one gene that makes sickle hemoglobin. But the other half of the equation, the beta thalassemia gene, produces either poorly functioning hemoglobin or none at all. In this situation, the majority—if not all—of the resulting hemoglobin is sickle hemoglobin.

So, sickle cell disease results not only from the inheritance of two sickle hemoglobin genes, but also from one sickle hemoglobin gene combined with another abnormal hemoglobin gene. While certain genetic differences mark each of these syndromes, the resulting symptoms are quite similar.

There are other types of sickle cell disease that are rarer: SO^{Arab}, SD^{Punjab} or $SD^{LosAngeles}$, and others.

What does the sickle hemoglobin do to cause sickling?

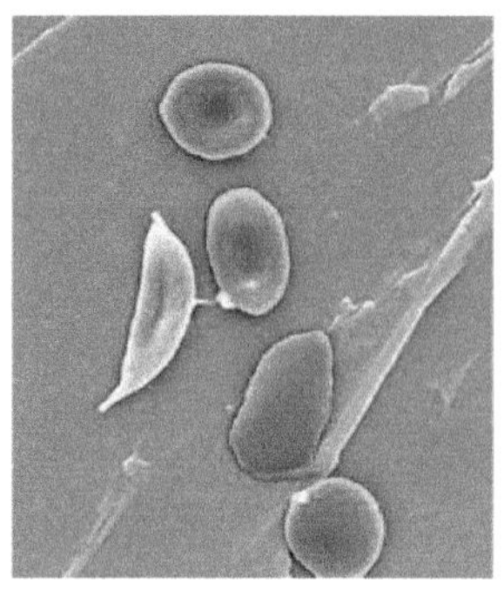

A normal red blood cell is round and soft, like a jelly donut. Red blood cells make up about 40%-45% of a person's blood and live for 120 days. A sickled red cell is shaped like a crescent moon, or a banana, or the farming tool called a sickle. Loss of oxygen is the most common trigger for the red blood cell to change shape.

Other reasons are dehydration or buildup of body acid.

What happens inside the red blood cell?

Hemoglobin normally floats around as separate molecules. Sickle hemoglobin stacks up (polymerizes) and makes long solid sticks that change the shape of the red blood cell.

Why does sickle cell disease make eyes yellow?

Jaundice is a sign of the breakdown of sickle red blood cells, and jaundiced eyes can be a baseline characteristic of people with sickle cell. The yellow color will be more intense as the red blood cells break down more quickly or if you do not drink enough fluids. It is not contagious, but some children become very self-conscious about jaundice.

What can I do to prevent sickle cell pain?

Vaso-occlusive pain, unpredictable severe pain which is a hallmark symptom of sickle cell disease, sometimes happens for no apparent reason. Some people with sickle cell disease report an early warning sensation before the pain.

Sometimes vaso-occlusive pain can be triggered by dehydration, exhaustion, infection, low oxygen, emotional stress, change of weather or chilled skin.

Things you can do for yourself to help avoid pain:

- Drink more fluids to prevent dehydration.
- When you notice that a trigger for pain is coming along, drink more fluids!
- Always drink more fluids when the weather changes and when the weather is very hot.
- Avoid common triggers like exhaustion from too much exercise, or exhaustion from poor sleeping habits; get plenty of rest and stick to a moderate activity level.
- Avoid triggers such as getting chilled after swimming—get a towel and dry yourself quickly.

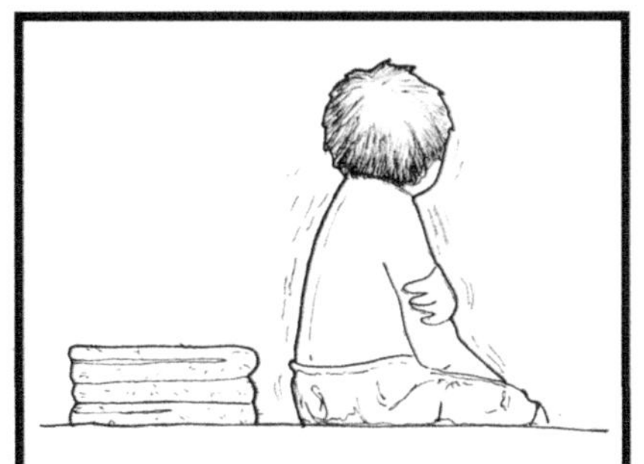

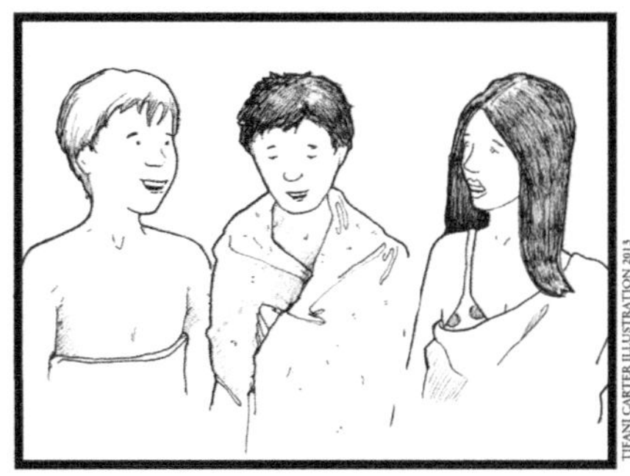

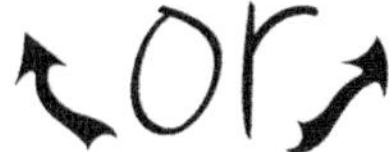

Exercise? Yes!
Staying active with sickle cell disease

Many people are mistaken and think that having sickle cell disease means they should engage in no physical activity. This is not true! Exercise can actually help blood flow and help

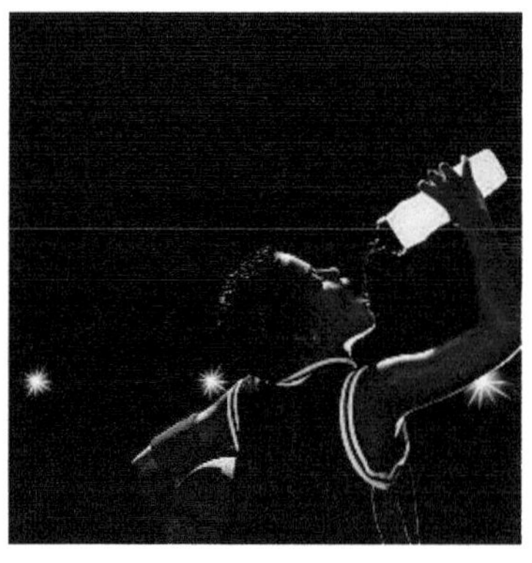

reduce crises or complications. You can stay active by choosing light to moderate types of physical activity: yoga, walking, swimming in a heated pool, volleyball, shooting basketballs. Avoid heavy joint impact like you would experience on a trampoline. Plan time to rest during and after exercise—rest breaks every twenty minutes are probably a good idea. Remember to drink lots of liquids, and don't push it too hard! Listen to your body.

Treatments at home

One way to remember the things you can do at home to help prevent sickle cell pain problems is the word FARMS:

Fluids: drinking a lot of fluids can help prevent red blood cells from sickling.

Air: get enough oxygen by taking deep breaths. Avoid conditions in which there is low oxygen, such as at high altitudes (over about 8,000 feet or about 2,500 meters). If you have asthma, be sure to treat it properly so that you do not have trouble breathing.

Rest/relaxation: take a rest break for a few minutes if you are playing or working vigorously. Build in breaks to relax if you are having a lot of emotional stress.

Medications/medical care: take medicines as prescribed by your doctors. See your doctors for regular check-ups, not just when you have pain or fever, so that problems can be detected early or even prevented. Ask questions about what else you can do to help yourself take care of your sickle cell disease.

Situations/support: avoid situations that can cause problems for your sickle cell disease: avoid getting chilled by wet clothing. Pay attention to the weather forecast and bring an umbrella if rain is likely. Friends might remind you to take a bottle of water with you when you are going out to play ball.

History of Sickle Cell Disease

The story of Walter Clement Noel

Sickle cell disease was first described to the Western world in Chicago, Illinois, about 100 years ago.

Walter Clement Noel finished his education in Grenada, a small island nation in the southeastern Caribbean Sea, and he wanted to continue to learn so he could become a dentist. He found out that Chicago was one of the few places that would train black men in dentistry.

His mother was worried about letting him go to Chicago. Why? Because it was more than 2,500 miles away, and he would be a foreigner in a big city. She heard that Chicago had beaches but that the sun was not as warm as in Grenada, and sometimes it was windy and snowy. But Walter was determined. He applied to the Chicago College of Dental Surgery and was accepted. His mother wrote a letter to the head of the dental school, asking him to look out for Walter.

Walter took a ship from Grenada to America. The trip took a week. He landed at Ellis Island, near the Statue of Liberty in New York Harbor on September 14, 1904, and made his way to Chicago. He started dental school very close to where the Illinois Medical District is today.

While in dental school, Walter got sick several times with strange pains. Sometimes his legs or his back hurt, and the doctors thought it was arthritis. Sometimes his chest hurt, and the doctors thought it was an infection in his lungs. Cold weather brought on more of these problems, and the pains became especially bad in the severe winter of 1905. His doctors could not figure out what was causing his problems, but they gave him morphine to help ease the pain.

One young doctor, Ernest E. Irons, had the bright idea to do a new test on Walter's blood.

He looked at a thin layer of Walter's blood under a microscope. Dr. Irons was very surprised to find "cells of an unusual elongated shape" and showed them to his professor, James B. Herrick. They did not know why Walter's cells looked this way, but they realized it was something new and not just arthritis or pneumonia. Dr. Herrick wrote a medical paper in 1910 describing this new disease. Other doctors began to recognize it in their patients experiencing similar symptoms when they looked under the microscope at their blood. They named it sickle cell disease, because the long shape and sharp pointed tips of the red blood cells reminded them of a farming tool called a sickle.

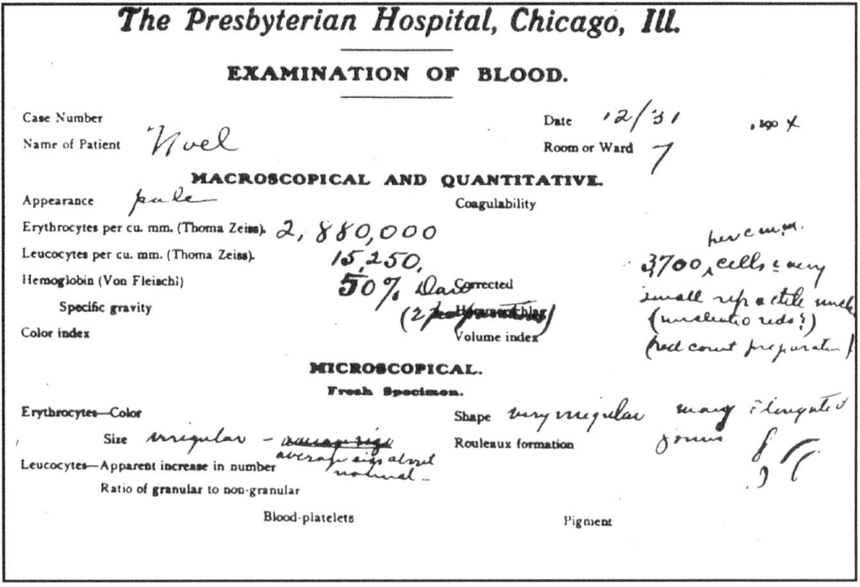

The Presbyterian Hospital, Chicago, Ill.

EXAMINATION OF BLOOD.

Case Number

Date 12/31, 190

Name of Patient Noel

Room or Ward 7

MACROSCOPICAL AND QUANTITATIVE.

Appearance pale

Coagulability

Erythrocytes per cu. mm. (Thoma Zeiss). 2,880,000

Leucocytes per cu. mm. (Thoma Zeiss). 15,250

Hemoglobin (Von Fleischl) 50%

Corrected

Specific gravity

Volume index

Color index

per cu. mm. 3700 cells

MICROSCOPICAL.

Fresh Specimen.

Erythrocytes—Color

Shape very irregular many elongated forms

Size irregular – average size almost normal –

Rouleaux formation

Leucocytes—Apparent increase in number

Ratio of granular to non-granular

Blood-platelets

Pigment

What happened to Walter Clement Noel? Over time, he learned that staying warm and drinking a lot of liquids kept his body stronger and helped him avoid some of the painful episodes. He studied hard, and the head of the dental school helped him catch up on the work he missed each time he was hospitalized. He graduated from dental school in 1907. The new Dr. Noel went back to Grenada on another ocean steamship voyage and set up his dental practice. Since the very first recognized case, people have been overcoming sickle cell disease with the support of family, such as Walter Noel's proud mother, and friends, such as the head of the Chicago College of Dental Surgery.

The origin of sickle cell disease in Africa

The majority of sickle cell cases have historically been found within the black population, with the highest number of known cases today found in Africa, making it likely that the very first case of the disease occurred in Africa.

African tribal populations did know of a disease that caused terrible pain. They named the disease in their own languages. Many tribal names describe a painful condition with names like "body chewing" or "body biting." Other names seem to copy or imitate the cries and moans heard from people suffering from the disease.

However, the first known reports of sickle cell disease did not come from Africa. This is probably due to several reasons:

1. The symptoms of sickle cell disease were similar to those of other common tropical diseases in Africa, so tribal populations probably treated those early cases of sickle cell disease like it was something else. Most people born in Africa with sickle cell disease before 1900 died as babies or young children and were typically not seen by doctors.
2. African tribal populations did not publish medical papers that the global scientific community could read and learn from. So while they knew about this pain-causing disease, they didn't share that information with other doctors in other parts of the world until the 1870s when the first reports of this disease appeared in African medical literature.
3. Tribal populations in Africa did not have microscopes to be able to look closely at blood and see the sickle-shaped blood cells of someone who has sickle cell disease until the late 1800s.

Understanding Your CBC Lab Results

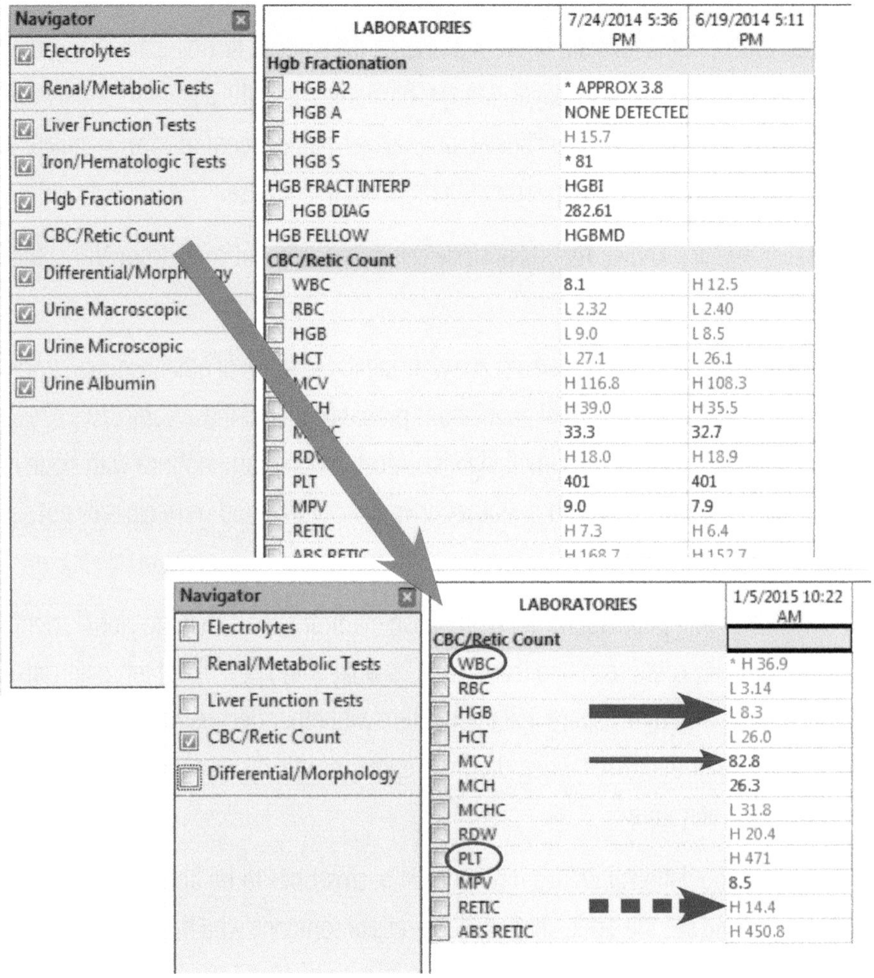

Navigator
- Electrolytes
- Renal/Metabolic Tests
- Liver Function Tests
- Iron/Hematologic Tests
- Hgb Fractionation
- CBC/Retic Count
- Differential/Morph[illegible]gy
- Urine Macroscopic
- Urine Microscopic
- Urine Albumin

LABORATORIES	7/24/2014 5:36 PM	6/19/2014 5:11 PM
Hgb Fractionation		
HGB A2	* APPROX 3.8	
HGB A	NONE DETECTEC	
HGB F	H 15.7	
HGB S	* 81	
HGB FRACT INTERP	HGBI	
HGB DIAG	282.61	
HGB FELLOW	HGBMD	
CBC/Retic Count		
WBC	8.1	H 12.5
RBC	L 2.32	L 2.40
HGB	L 9.0	L 8.5
HCT	L 27.1	L 26.1
MCV	H 116.8	H 108.3
[illegible]CH	H 39.0	H 35.5
M[illegible]C	33.3	32.7
RD[illegible]	H 18.0	H 18.9
PLT	401	401
MPV	9.0	7.9
RETIC	H 7.3	H 6.4
ABS RETIC	H 168.7	H 152.7

Navigator
- Electrolytes
- Renal/Metabolic Tests
- Liver Function Tests
- CBC/Retic Count
- Differential/Morphology

LABORATORIES	1/5/2015 10:22 AM
CBC/Retic Count	
WBC	* H 36.9
RBC	L 3.14
HGB	L 8.3
HCT	L 26.0
MCV	82.8
MCH	26.3
MCHC	L 31.8
RDW	H 20.4
PLT	H 471
MPV	8.5
RETIC	H 14.4
ABS RETIC	H 450.8

What are the key parts of the blood counts (CBC and reticulocyte count) that I need to understand when reviewing my lab results?

- The thickest arrow is on <u>Hemoglobin (Hgb or Hb)</u>. Lower numbers mean more severe anemia.

- The dashed line shows the Reticulocyte percentage. Higher numbers mean more red blood cells are newly produced.
- The thin arrow is on Mean Cell Volume (MCV). Higher numbers mean bigger red blood cells. Higher MCV is one of the helpful effects of hydroxyurea treatment.
- WBC is white blood cell count. Higher numbers mean inflammation or infection, or other stress to the body.
- Plt is Platelet count. The platelet count can change in many sickle cell conditions.

The lab sheet lists so many results as abnormal. How do I interpret my own CBC and reticulocyte results?

Having sickle cell disease makes many of your CBC results fall outside the ranges for people without any blood disorder. But looking over your CBC and reticulocyte results with your doctor can show you that many results always are the same when you are doing well. These are your own "baseline" CBC results.

Do the CBC and reticulocyte results measure pain?

It is important to know that pain cannot be measured with the CBC, the reticulocyte count, or with any other blood test available (as of 2015). You can still have sickle cell pain or other medical problems while your CBC and reticulocyte counts are "normal" for you, meaning they are at your baseline.

What if the CBC and reticulocyte results are <u>not</u> at my baseline?

Interpreting why CBC or reticulocyte results are <u>not</u> at baseline in people with sickle cell can be very complicated. Not every doctor learns these skills. That is one of the biggest reasons why you should see a hematologist, or another doctor with a lot of experience treating sickle cell disease. Your hematologist can advise you on what to do and what treatment options are available to get your CBC and reticulocyte results back to your baseline.

Treatment Options

Pain, pain, go away!

Sickle cell disease can cause pain. Generally, pain affects the long bones, the spine, and the ribcage. Sometimes it is an ache that is not too bad. Sometimes the pain can be more intense and needs medicine. Sometimes the pain is really too much to handle at home and you have to go to the hospital for treatment.

One common way to think about your pain medication is to imagine a staircase that organizes how you select pain medications. When the pain is higher, you need to climb to a higher level of the staircase and add on more pain medications. When the pain gets better, you can go to a lower level of pain medications.

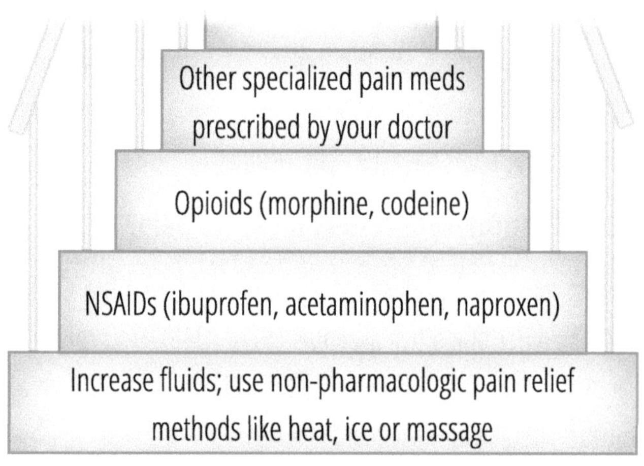

Blood transfusion (adapted from www.redcrossblood.org)

Many problems with sickle cell disease can be managed through blood transfusions.

What is a blood transfusion? How does it work?

Approximately 5 million people per year in the U.S. receive blood transfusions. A blood transfusion is a safe, common procedure in which you receive blood through an intravenous (IV) line inserted into one of your blood vessels. Through this line, you receive red blood cells that do not sickle.

A nurse will bring in a bag of blood that has been specially selected for you. The bag will hang on a pole near your hospital bed and a tube will be inserted into the bag. Then the blood can travel from the bag, through the IV and into your blood vessels. The procedure usually takes two to four hours, depending on how much blood you need. Most of the time, you will not feel any discomfort when the blood goes in. Nurses and others will make sure you feel okay during the transfusion. A nurse keeps an eye on your temperature and blood pressure and looks to make sure there is no rash or other signs of an allergic reaction.

When does a person with sickle cell get a blood transfusion?

A transfusion can provide better oxygen for a short time when anemia is very severe or when your body is going through severe stress. These are some of the sickle cell problems that might require a transfusion:

- aplastic crisis
- acute spleen problems
- acute chest syndrome
- severe illness
- preparation for surgery or general anesthesia

Some patients get transfusions every month for years to reduce the effects of sickle red blood cells. Regular transfusions might also be used if there are long-term problems with major organs like the heart, lungs or kidneys. An abnormal transcranial Doppler scan can also make regular transfusions necessary in an effort to prevent a stroke.

Hydroxyurea

What is hydroxyurea?

Hydroxyurea is a medicine that is taken daily to help make severe sickle cell disease become a milder disease. Hydroxyurea is not a treatment for pain once a pain episode has started. It is not a cure for sickle cell, but it has been used to control symptoms since the 1990s. Hydroxyurea cannot cure sickle cell disease completely, but it can make sickle cell disease less severe by making your red blood cells less likely to sickle so they can move through small blood vessels more easily. Talk to your hematology doctor about whether hydroxyurea is right for you.

How does hydroxyurea help people with sickle cell disease?

Hydroxyurea can raise your level of fetal hemoglobin and increase the size of your red blood cells—both of these effects will make the red blood cell less likely to sickle. Hydroxyurea also makes the red blood cells less sticky so that they move through small blood vessels more easily. In addition, hydroxyurea helps block some of the abnormal properties of other blood cells and blood vessels, which also helps blood flow more easily.

Hydroxyurea is helpful

Hydroxyurea usually prevents about half of a patient's problems with pain episodes and acute chest syndrome. This means fewer blood transfusions and longer periods of time between hospitalizations. People on hydroxyurea have fewer unpredictable absences from school or work, which helps them fulfill their career goals.

Hydroxyurea can also prevent some priapism, painful erections of the penis lasting longer than four hours. Sickle cell patients who take hydroxyurea tend to live longer and maintain good brain function longer, and children on hydroxyurea gain weight better.

What to check while you are on hydroxyurea

If you take hydroxyurea, you should have frequent blood tests in order to monitor your blood counts. Taking hydroxyurea might cause a risk to a fetus if the mother or father is taking hydroxyurea at the time of conception, so an acceptable method of birth control is necessary while taking hydroxyurea.

Curing sickle cell disease with stem cell transplant

At the time of this writing, the only cure for sickle cell disease is a transplant of bone marrow or other stem cells. This method is not yet ready for every single person with sickle cell disease, but a lot progress is being made. Over 600 people have had transplants for sickle cell disease.

What is bone marrow?

The soft spongy stuff in the middle of bones is called bone marrow. Marrow contains blood stem cells, which produce the cells of the blood: red blood cells that carry oxygen, white blood cells that fight infection and platelets that stop bleeding. Some people call the marrow the "blood factory."

What is the connection between bone marrow and sickle cell disease?

Sickle genes tell the bone marrow stem cells to make abnormal red blood cells that contain sickle hemoglobin instead of normal hemoglobin. It makes sense that to cure sickle cell requires correction of the bone marrow stem cells.

If the marrow donor has a different set of genes, like sickle trait or no sickle gene at all, then that donor's marrow stem cells makes red blood cells that will not sickle.

How is the bone marrow donated? Is it surgery?

It is surgery, but not with a scalpel. Marrow cells are collected from the pelvic bone (between the spine and where a hip pocket would be) using a special needle. Donors receive general anesthesia so no pain is experienced during the marrow extraction, which takes about two hours. The donor ends up with large bandage on the area. Within a week of donating, most donors can to return to work, school and many regular activities. The donor's marrow grows back within a few weeks.

Are blood stem cells only found in the bone marrow?

Some stem cells are also found in the blood, especially in a newborn baby's blood. These stem cells can also be used for transplants.

The placenta and umbilical cord are attached to the baby in the womb, but they are then set aside after the baby is born. Cord blood can be collected from the placenta and umbilical cord after birth without any harm to the baby.

Blood stem cells are also present in small quantities in the blood of an adult. Donors receive daily injections of a medicine called filgrastim for four days before and on the first day of the collection to increase the number of stem cells in the bloodstream. The blood stem cells can be removed by running the adult donor's blood through a filtering machine. The remaining blood flows back into the donor. The donor's blood stem cells will grow back.

How do the stem cells get into the recipient? Is it surgery?

Bone marrow transplant is not surgery. The blood stem cells are put in a bag that looks a lot like a blood transfusion bag. The cells go through an intravenous line into the transplant recipient, just like a blood transfusion. The stem cells find their way to the bone marrow space and start to grow there.

What does HLA mean?

Human leukocyte antigen (HLA) typing is used to match patients and donors for blood stem cell transplants. HLA are proteins, or markers, found on most cells in your body. Your immune system uses these markers to recognize which cells belong in your body and which do not.

How successful is bone marrow transplantation for sickle cell disease?

Bone marrow transplantation is mostly performed on children severely affected by sickle cell disease with donors who are an HLA-matched brother or sister. Hundreds of transplants have been done this way. The first transplants for sickle cell were performed in the early 1990s but had some problems. Since then doctors have adjusted the transplant procedures to make a special package for sickle cell patients. Starting around 2000, these new transplants have had success rates of more than 95% for children with a donor who is an HLA-matched brother or sister. Despite this success, there is some chance of graft rejection, which means that you have a transplant but it is not successful in curing your sickle cell disease. There is also some chance of death.

How much of the sickle cell disease will be cured by transplant?

Anemia and jaundice should go away, and there should be no new problems with pain, acute chest syndrome, priapism, spleen or other pain- related problems. Long-term pain might take six months to go away completely after a transplant. Growth and development will probably improve, and no new strokes should occur.

However, organs already damaged by sickle cell disease will probably not heal completely. Weakness or other loss of function from previous strokes will not go away, but prior damage to kidneys, lungs or hip joints could improve.

What are possible side effects of the transplant?

Side effects of bone marrow transplants depend on the type of preparation used for the transplant.

- The strong chemotherapy medicines used in most transplants can make it difficult for patients to go through puberty or eventually have children. Their hair probably will fall out, but it will grow back. Chemotherapy can temporarily cause vomiting, but there are good medicines to control it. Infection or organ damage can cause death.
- Radiation therapy can have similar effects to chemotherapy. Immunosuppressant therapy has different side effects, mainly causing the body to be wide-open to infections.
- GVHD is sometimes a mild and treatable condition, but it can also become a long-term problem that might be worse than sickle cell disease in some people. GVHD can also cause death. GVHD can occur with any type of transplant, but is more likely

when the donor is not perfect HLA match.

- There is a higher risk of bad side effects if a patient was in very poor health before the transplant. To check for side effects, transplant doctors usually will schedule a lot of follow-up appointments.

The newest transplant method for sickle cell is the non-ablative approach. It also is called *partial mixed chimerism*. With this method, enough donor marrow is transplanted to the patient to produce normal red blood cells. The better red blood cells produced by the donor marrow have a longer lifespan than sickle red blood cells, which will allow the healthy cells to eventually become the majority of the circulating red blood cells.

It is believed that we do not need to wipe out all of the marrow cells to put in the blood stem cells from a sibling to correct sickle cell disease. When less than full doses of chemo or radiation are used for transplant, the end result is often a mixture of patient and donor stem cells in the bone marrow. This mixture of stem cells then makes the mixture of blood cells circulating throughout the body.

Do you know that people talk about marrow and blood like they talk about fruit trees? The cells that produce these blood cells are called "stem cells" because they are like the stem of a plant.

Fruit tree	**Marrow**
the stem	marrow cells
leaves, flowers, and fruit	red blood cells, white blood cells, and platelets
the stem grows leaves, flowers, and fruit	marrow stem cells produce red blood cells, white blood cells, and platelets

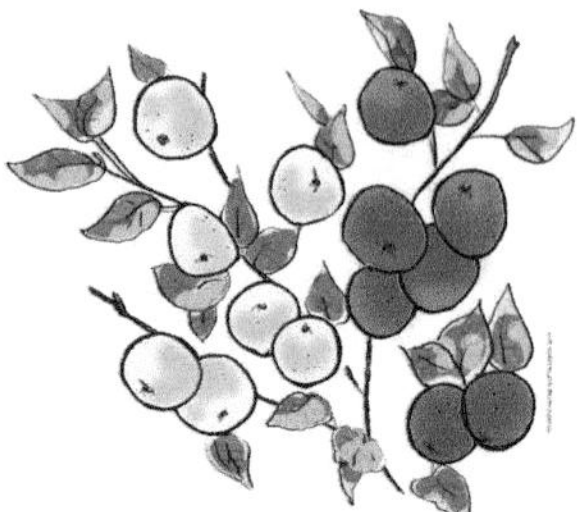

What is a Health Passport?

Why should I keep track of my medical records? How do I do it?

Every time you see your doctors or go to the hospital, they keep detailed notes in writing or on computers about your health history—these are your medical records. Doctors look up your records to remember what happened to you in the past so that they can understand better how to treat you today. Your family probably has been keeping track of your medical records since you were born.

Many families choose one or more of these options:

- Keep copies of all medical records in a notebook or folder.
- Write notes in a notebook and bring it to all medical appointments.
- Keep a copy of just the most important papers that summarize your medical history.
- Memorize the most important information in your medical history.

Here are three new options you can use from your computer or a mobile device:

1. Use mobile apps like VoiceCrisisAlert or SiKL that can be downloaded from http://crisisvoice.com and https://itunes.apple.com/gb/app/sikl/id640126148?mt=8.
2. Use a web-based Personal Medical Record like HealthVault or Kaiser's My Health Manager.
3. Use the Patient Portal feature of your doctor's electronic medical record. By 2016, most American hospital systems will offer this option.

All of your medical records will stay together as long as you keep going to the same doctor and hospital. When you go to a new doctor or hospital, one of the first things you will be asked is to remember all of your medical history until they can get a copy of the medical records from your other doctor or hospital.

You can offer to help track your medical records as you grow older. When you become an adult, you will be expected to keep track of your own medical records.

Another time that you might need to have your medical records is when you travel—to camp, on a long field trip, or other trips. For this reason, a medical summary is sometimes nicknamed a health passport because it is an important set of papers, just like a passport is an important document to prove your citizenship when you travel. Go to page 37 to find a health passport where you can fill in all your own medical information.

What happens if I do not have medical records or a health passport?

Without your medical records, you may get incorrect or delayed treatment, including:

- a duplicate test or injection
- a medicine that triggers an allergic reaction
- a transfusion that triggers a transfusion reaction
- a waste of time trying medication doses or treatments again that did not work for you in the first place
- delay while the doctors or hospital ask you to remember your medical history and request medical records from the other doctors or hospital

Hobby & Career Choices

Live every day to the fullest and prepare for a life into adulthood. Preparation should be made for work, marriage, hobbies and meaningful contributions to society. Education and skills are very important.

Jobs that require heavy activity or working outdoors in bad weather are not good choices for people with sickle cell disease. Professional sports that involve endurance performance are not likely to be good choices either. Aim for indoor jobs, flexible schedules or white-collar jobs. You will probably need good grades and college or a professional education. Performing arts can be a good choice. Some famous musicians had sickle cell disease.

Real-life careers of people with sickle cell disease

Lawyer
Physician
Psychologist
Minister
Teacher
Gospel singer
Electrical engineer
Business owner
Vice president of a multinational computer software company
Public health policy-maker at the Centers for Disease Control
NASA engineer
Clinical research nurse
Daycare center owner
Accountant
Journalist
Computer programmer
Professor
Disc jockey
Health education policy-maker at the National Institutes of Health
Parent/grandparent

Miles Davis, famous jazz musician, lived with sickle cell disease.Widely considered one of the most influential musicians of the 20th century, Miles Davis (1926-1991), with his musical groups, was at the forefront of several major developments in jazz music,

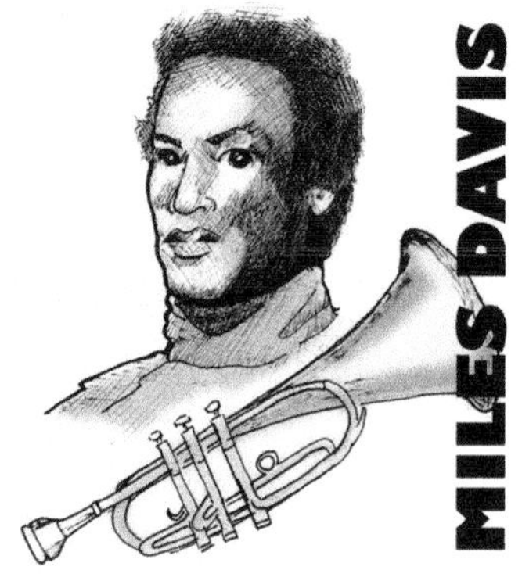

including bebop, cool jazz, hard bop, modal jazz, and jazz fusion.

Miles Davis had sickle cell disease. Sickle cell caused him a lot of pain and hip joint problems, and he underwent hip replacements starting in 1976 when he was just 50 years old. But it did not stop this nine-time Grammy Award-winning trumpet player and songwriter from playing great music for more than five decades and acting as a catalyst for other musicians to bring forth new types of music.

Source: "Miles Davis." Bio. A&E Television Networks, 2015. Web. 08 Jan. 2015. Retrieved from http://www.biography.com/people/miles-davis-9267992.

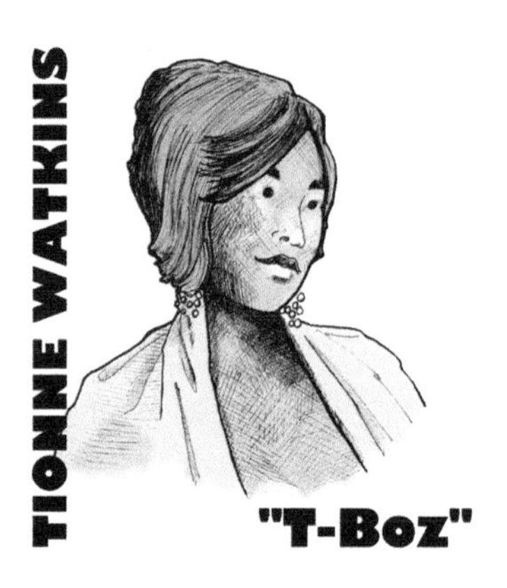

Despite hospitalizations at an early age due to sickle cell disease, Tionne "T-Boz" Watkins (born in 1970) grew up to become a four-time Grammy Award-winning musician as a member of the successful R&B trio, TLC. Despite battling sickle cell disease all her life and overcoming a brain tumor in her 30s, Watkins is now in her mid-40s and has enjoyed the success of the TLC musical group and her own solo singing career, participated in a reality-television show, published a book of her own poetry and even owned a children's clothing boutique. Watkins became an official spokesperson of the Sickle Cell Disease Association of America in 1996 and serves as a strong role model for others with sickle cell anemia and other blood disorders.

Source: "Tionne "T-Boz" Watkins." Bio. A&E Television Networks, 2015. Web. 08 Jan. 2015. Retrieved from http://www.biography.com/people/tionne-t-boz-watkins-21306077.

Tips for Learning to Live Well with SCD

Avoid infection: five tips to help prevent infections

Common illnesses, such as the flu, can quickly become dangerous for a person with sickle cell disease. The best defense is to take simple steps to help prevent infections.

Hand washing

Washing your hands is one of the best ways to help prevent getting an infection. People with sickle cell disease, their family and other caretakers should wash their hands with soap and clean water many times each day. If you don't have soap and water, you can use gel hand cleaners with alcohol in them.

Times to wash your hands:

BEFORE

- Making food
- Eating

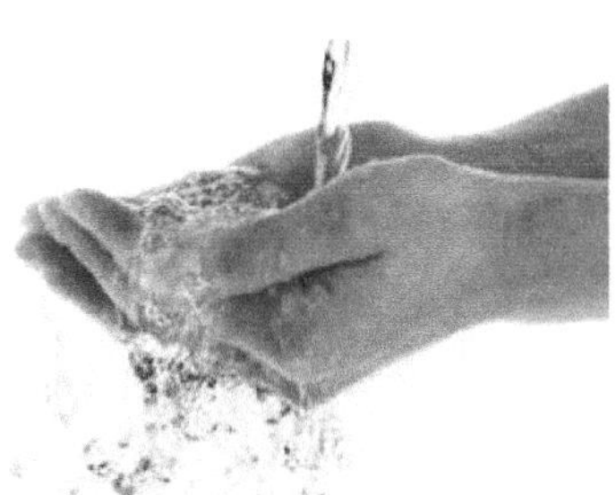

AFTER

- Using the bathroom
- Blowing your nose, coughing, or sneezing
- Shaking hands
- Touching people or things that can carry germs, such as:
    - Diapers or a child who has used the toilet
    - Food that is not cooked (raw meat, raw eggs, or unwashed vegetables)
    - Animals or animal waste

- Trash
- A sick person

Food safety

Salmonella, a bacteria in some foods, can be especially harmful to children with sickle cell disease. How to stay safe when cooking and eating:

- Wash hands, cutting boards, counters, knives, and other utensils after they touch uncooked foods.
- Wash vegetables and fruit well before eating them.
- Cook meat until it is well done. The juices should run clear and there should be no pink inside.
- Do not eat raw or undercooked eggs. Raw eggs might be hiding in home-made hollandaise sauce, Caesar and other homemade salad dressings, tiramisu, homemade ice cream, homemade mayonnaise, cookie dough and frostings.
- Do not eat raw or unpasteurized milk or other dairy products. Make sure these foods have a label that says they are "pasteurized."

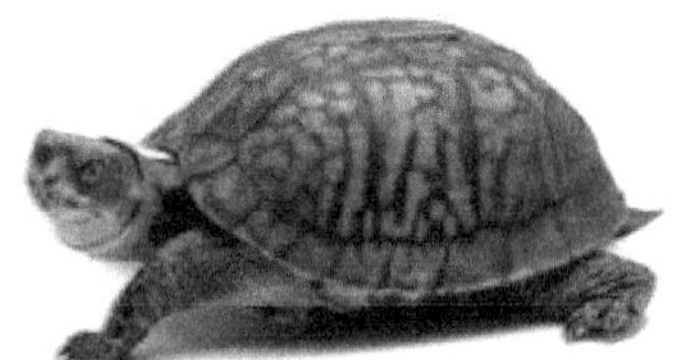

Reptiles

Salmonella can also be carried by reptiles. Make sure children stay away from turtles, snakes and lizards.

Vaccines

Vaccines are a great way to prevent many serious infections. Children with sickle cell disease should get all the regular childhood vaccines, plus a few extra.

The extra ones are:

- Flu vaccine every year after six months of age.

- A pneumococcal vaccine (called 23-valent pneumococcal vaccine) at two and five years of age.
- Meningococcal vaccine (talk to your doctor about the new 2014 recommendations for this vaccine).

Source: www.cdc.gov/meningococcal/outbreaks/vaccine-serogroupb.html

- Conjugated pneumococcal vaccine PCV-13 (at least once).

Adults should have the flu vaccine every year, as well as the pneumococcal vaccine and any others recommended by a doctor.

Penicillin

Take penicillin (or another antibiotic prescribed by a doctor) every day until at least five years of age.

Why is it important to see my hematologist for regular check-ups, not just when I'm sick?

Preventive care

Visit your hematologist regularly so that you can catch problems BEFORE they make you sick!

- Immunizations or antibiotics to prevent infection
- Screening tests for early detection and preventive care—stroke, vision loss, lung, heart, and kidney
- Hydroxyurea
- Chronic transfusion
- Iron overload

Specialty care

Your hematologist is an expert at helping people with sickle cell disease, and they know how to help you feel better when you are in pain and how to stay away from things that could make you sick.

- Reduce triggers for pain—menses, sleep apnea, asthma, gallstones
- Pain management—prescription pain medication, multiple modalities
- Hydroxyurea
- Chronic transfusion
- Iron overload
- Bone marrow/stem cell transplantation

A medical advocate and a medical home

Think of your hematologist as your sickle cell coach. They keep track of all your symptoms, health history, vaccine records and past medical treatments to help you make the best decisions and keep you healthy, just like a coach makes sure that every practice is safe, that the players are working together as a team and that the team has everything it needs to win.

- Coordinate care—watch out for overlapping and contradicting treatment
- Medical forms and counseling about rights: Americans with Disabilities Act, FMLA, etc.
- Plan for surgery (do not consent to general anesthesia without medical clearance)—gallbladder, hip, tonsil, dental, spleen, port, bypass
- Baseline labs and X-rays (avoid or reduce repeat testing)

Supervision of potential medication allergies

Your hematologist will monitor any reactions or side-effects you have to medicines and other treatments, so you know what to stay away from.

- Transfusion reactions and alloantibodies—these can be as life-threatening as medication allergies
- Medical summary

Learning about resources

Your hematologist can show you where to find trustworthy information for taking good care of yourself.

- New treatments
- Community events and support resources—summer camp, parties, conferences and scholarships
- Personal advocacy and empowerment
- Political action

The opportunity to help others

There are lots of kids just like you who have sickle cell disease and experience pain and frustration at times. Sometimes it helps people when they can talk to someone who really understands what they are going through because they've gone through it too. Talk to your hematologist if you want to help other kids with sickle cell disease or get involved with new research.

- Support groups
- 1:1 Discussions
- Participate in research

Emergency Guide: When to See the Doctor

It is very important that every person with sickle cell disease have a plan for how to get help immediately, at any hour, if there is a problem. Be sure to find a place that will have access to your medical records or bring a copy that you have handy at home with you.

Go to an emergency room or call your doctor right away for:

- Fever above 101° F
- Difficulty breathing
- Chest pain
- Abdominal (belly) swelling
- Severe headache
- Sudden weakness or loss of feeling and movement
- Seizure
- Painful erection of the penis that lasts more than 1 hour
- Any sudden problem with vision

Stories From Sickle Cell Patients Like You

"I found out about the sickle cell disease when I was four years old. Before we knew what the disease was, I had had several mild crises, such as pain and swelling.

When I was six years old, I had my first violent crisis. It was then we discovered why I was suffering so much. After that, from September 2006 to April 2010, I was in the hospital every three months suffering many crises and taking continuous doses of morphine, Tramal, Tylex, aspirin, Lisador, dipyrone, Alivium, and so on. It was a cocktail to ease the intense pain that was crossing my whole body, not to mention unaccountable blood transfusions.

Every crisis was accompanied with pneumonia. During this period, I also underwent surgery for a hernia and a gallbladder. I could not do any type of physical exertion. I could not run, jump, ride a bike, nor have any kind of fun. Everything resulted in returning to the hospital.

In April 2010, I was taken to the "Holy" Boldrini Center in São Paolo, Brazil. At the first consultation I was started on Hydrea, a wonderful medicine that saved my life. It completely changed my way of life.

Since then, I have never felt any pain. I am another person. I was able to develop myself both physically and mentally. I still have be in treatment every three months, but I am living another life. I'm so happy. I do physical education at school, ride my bike, run and do everything, within my limits, of course. My eating habits have changed 100% and they are much healthier. Today I can truly be thankful for my treatment. I appreciate all the attention, care and affection that I have received and which has changed my life.

Thanks, Boldrini family."

Herick – 12 years old

"My name is Samara Cristina. A few days after my birth I started getting sick with fever and infection. I started taking antibiotics and every ten days the antibiotics were changed.

For months my mom and I suffered because we did not know what I had. Because my mother did not know what I had, nothing was resolved. Finally she talked to my dad, and they decided to pay for a private doctor to find out what I really had.

When my mother took me to the private doctor, he asked us to take some tests. I did them. When I went back to the doctor he said that I had sickle cell anemia and explained what this was to my mother. The doctor explained that he was already suspicious that it was this disease since I was anemic, and he had already treated a boy with the same symptoms.

I started the treatments when I was one year and two months old. When I was seven, my mother told me what I had. It was sickle cell anemia, and she said that I could lead a normal life, but I would have limitations.

Today I'm 18 years old. I have finished my studies and I plan to go to college."

Elvis had sickle cell disease in Brazil. He lived with frequent pain and recurrent priapism. He also had leg ulcers. He recalls many sleepless nights because of sickle cell pain. When he was 38, his brother donated bone marrow for a transplant. This made him one of the oldest people with sickle cell to have a BMT. He has been going around the country telling people about sickle cell disease.

Today he is 42 years old and doing well 4 years after his bone marrow transplant. Elvis said, "I never knew I could feel this good to live without sickle cell pain." His only medication is daily penicillin because of his functional asplenia. He is among the leaders of ABRADFAL, the Brazilian advocacy group for sickle cell disease. He stands up in international meetings to speak up for more services for sickle cell.

African Sickle Cell News & World Report Vol. 4 (1) Jan-Mar 2012

The Inheritance Game

What does it mean to inherit a sickle gene?

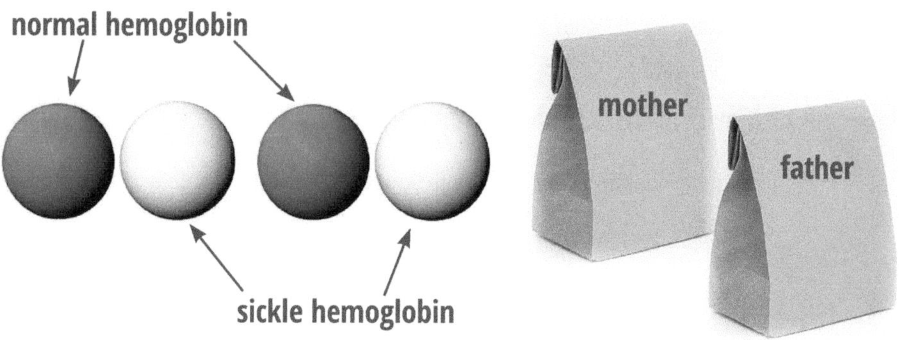

Because this is a genetic condition, whether somebody gets sickle cell disease or sickle trait depends on what genes you get from your parents. Here is a little game to demonstrate what it means to inherit a sickle gene.

The Inheritance Game

You will need:

- Four small balls that are the same except that they are different colors.
  For the instructions, we will pretend there are two blue balls and two white balls. If you do not have two colors of balls, you can use marbles or candies or pencils—any set of four things that come in two colors.
- Two bags that do not allow you to see what is inside.
  A paper lunch bag can be used. Label or decorate one bag "Mother" and one bag "Father."

Pretend that different balls stand for different genes; one type of ball (blue) stands for normal hemoglobin genes and another ball (white) for sickle hemoglobin genes. Every person has two genes for hemoglobin. A person with sickle trait has one normal hemoglobin gene and one sickle hemoglobin gene (one blue ball and one white ball).

1. If the mother has sickle trait, she has one normal and one sickle gene. Put one blue

and one white ball in the bag labeled "Mother."

2. If the father has sickle trait also, he has one normal and one sickle gene. Put one blue and one white ball in the bag labeled "Father."

3. When the mother and father have a baby, the baby gets one gene from the mother and one gene from the father—reach into the bag and pull one ball from each and see what genes the baby has now.

4. What kind of hemoglobin condition do these genes give this baby? Choices are:

- Normal hemoglobin (two blue balls)
- Sickle trait (one blue ball and one white ball)
- Sickle cell disease (two white balls)

That's right! You learned how a mother and a father's genes can give a baby a new genetic combination. So you see that this is one possible combination from this imaginary mother & father who both have sickle trait. Another baby from the same parents could have any of the other combinations of genes, because with every pregnancy there is a random chance of each gene combination.

Word Searches

Organs affected by sickle cell

Words to find: eye, brain, skin, spleen, shoulder, liver, placenta, kidney, lungs, hip, marrow

A	J	M	H	X	P	Y	U	A	X	L	I	L	V	N
R	T	S	S	R	E	D	L	U	O	H	S	U	X	O
F	R	N	S	K	P	F	M	C	C	X	I	N	A	Y
L	O	D	E	O	I	G	Q	L	N	T	R	G	M	C
H	S	W	W	C	H	G	I	B	J	W	A	S	Q	Y
F	X	L	Y	Q	A	V	W	N	G	A	J	C	E	N
L	J	F	V	U	E	L	Y	E	B	Z	E	N	A	X
O	L	L	C	R	W	D	P	E	T	R	D	F	K	C
L	U	D	T	D	M	Q	P	L	U	I	A	O	T	O
J	R	B	D	E	N	W	X	P	K	L	X	I	W	U
R	E	O	L	P	Y	Y	V	S	X	O	H	N	N	G
M	A	R	R	O	W	E	P	A	Q	W	X	X	B	Y
H	J	A	A	F	D	K	F	X	O	N	I	K	S	V
C	T	O	H	L	X	U	T	T	F	V	J	E	G	S
P	X	Z	A	U	N	A	P	X	O	W	H	P	T	V

Countries that have a lot of sickle cell patients

Words to find: Nigeria, Congo, Tanzania, Zambia, Uganda, Angola, Niger, Cameroon, India, Brazil, Togo, Sierra Leone

```
A C T B P G N N C R U A U Z L
L D H A J A I B M A Z L W W K
H N N T N G E L Q S Z O P O O
M W N A E Z I T C C E G A V G
T L G R G Z A E S N I N C M U
E F I P A U L N M N Y A O T D
M A H R E M W F I K C A S I B
E Y B S I E R R A A A Y U L B
Z J S N C E N O E L M L N F B
Y M D I C O N Q R B E F B D R
U I H G N K N E X Z R K D G E
A K W E F J Y G Y V O E X H M
E Z X R H A X B O N O G Q L Q
O S Z U W P E Y L E N X O S H
D N O I S D E K B O N Q R T C
```

Occupations of people with sickle cell

Words to find: lawyer, NASA engineer, physician, clinical researcher, nurse, psychologist, daycare owner, minister, accountant, Realtor, teacher, journalist, gospel singer, computer programmer

G	R	L	A	G	T	E	A	C	H	E	R	R	C	T
O	O	O	A	S	R	N	V	M	O	N	O	E	L	S
S	H	R	E	W	A	A	I	W	J	U	S	S	I	I
P	T	O	L	I	Y	N	N	F	Z	R	S	E	N	L
E	U	T	E	J	I	E	I	D	I	S	E	A	I	A
L	A	L	C	S	R	L	R	V	P	E	F	R	C	N
T	N	A	T	N	U	O	C	C	A	A	O	C	A	R
T	H	E	R	E	N	G	I	N	E	E	R	H	L	U
L	R	R	I	E	R	A	C	Y	A	D	P	E	J	O
P	S	Y	C	H	O	L	O	G	I	S	T	R	N	J
O	T	N	A	I	C	I	S	Y	H	P	O	U	O	T
F	Z	N	L	R	E	T	U	P	M	O	C	L	C	N
R	E	G	N	I	S	M	B	U	S	I	N	E	S	S
J	O	C	K	E	Y	H	T	L	A	E	H	S	I	X
F	G	E	P	R	O	G	R	A	M	M	E	R	D	N

Things that help with sickle cell pain

Words to find: friends, water, hot pack, music, movies, stories, coloring, knitting, phone, dreaming, prayer, games, poetry, breathing, sleep, massage, relaxation, acupuncture, bath, pets

G	C	C	I	D	Q	Z	I	M	D	A	K	E	Y	O
S	C	S	S	D	N	E	I	R	F	S	N	G	Z	H
S	E	O	M	P	K	P	E	L	E	W	I	A	P	Z
E	E	V	L	C	O	A	E	I	K	N	T	S	E	H
R	B	M	A	O	M	E	V	T	O	T	T	S	E	K
U	G	P	A	I	R	O	T	I	S	N	I	A	L	T
T	W	S	N	G	M	I	T	R	M	L	N	M	S	C
C	A	G	E	E	F	A	N	U	Y	C	G	M	L	A
N	T	R	I	I	X	Z	S	G	P	R	A	Y	E	R
U	E	Q	R	A	R	I	B	A	T	H	V	W	C	K
P	R	N	L	L	C	O	N	W	J	U	J	Y	Q	O
U	E	E	G	P	C	O	T	J	T	Q	J	Z	U	V
C	R	D	X	S	O	V	N	S	B	X	R	J	Q	H
A	M	P	D	C	V	J	P	J	G	Q	J	Q	X	O
B	R	E	A	T	H	I	N	G	E	N	O	H	P	T

My Health Passport
(Medical Information to Keep)

Name: ____

Date of Birth: ____

Sickle Cell Type: ____

Medical Record Number: ____

Allergies: ____

Medications: ____

Physician: ____

Phone number: ____

Complications: ____

Transfusions: ____

Transfusion problems or alloantibodies? yes/no

Blood bank that has my records: ____

Surgeries: ____

Pain Medications: ____

ER Pain Medications: ____

Where Does It Hurt?

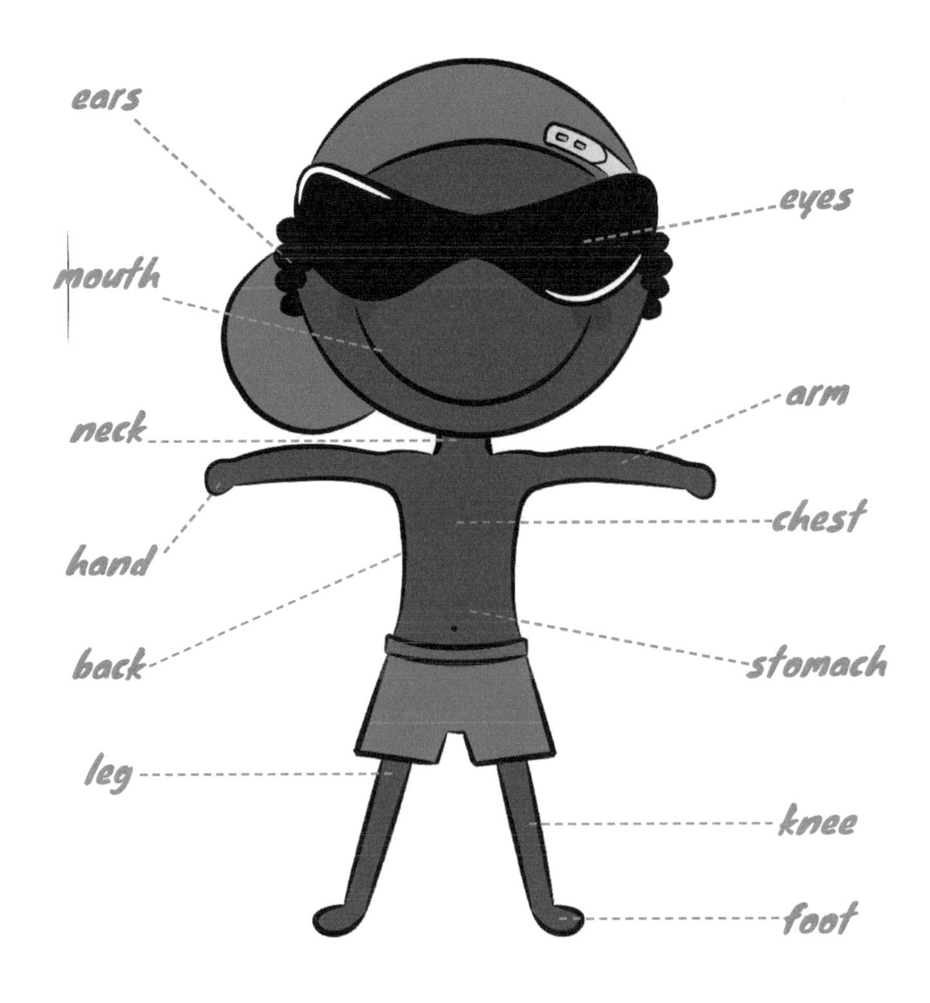

My Sickle Cell Journal

In this 18-month journal you can keep track of any pain you are feeling, side effects from medication or treatments, and any other concerns or questions you want to talk to your doctor about at your next visit.

Month: ______________________ My Health Summary: ______________

____

____

____

____

____

____

Month: ______________________ My Health Summary: ______________

____

____

____

____

____

____

Month: ______________________ My Health Summary: ______________

____

____

____

____

____

____

____

Month: ______________________ My Health Summary: ______________

Month: ______________________ My Health Summary: ______________

Month: ______________________ My Health Summary: ______________

Month: ______________________ My Health Summary: ______________

Month: ______________________ My Health Summary: ______________

Month: ______________________ My Health Summary: ______________

Month: ____________________ My Health Summary: ____________

Month: ____________________ My Health Summary: ____________

Month: ____________________ My Health Summary: ____________

Month: ______________________ My Health Summary: ______________

Month: ______________________ My Health Summary: ______________

Month: ______________________ My Health Summary: ______________

Month: ______________________ My Health Summary: ______________

Month: ______________________ My Health Summary: ______________

Month: ______________________ My Health Summary: ______________

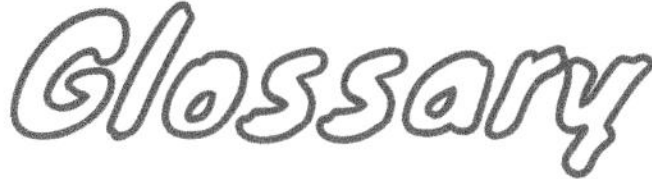

Acute Chest Syndrome—When sickled red blood cells block blood flow to the lungs. This can cause chest pain, shortness of breath, and cough. It is treated in the hospital with blood transfusions. It can be prevented with incentive spirometry (a "blow bottle").

Advocacy—Health advocacy supports and promotes patient's health care rights. Advocacy activities can also include working to enhance community health, and working to change government policies on making health care available, safe, and with high quality.

Anemia—A low red blood cell count. Anemia can be caused by many different events, including sickle cell disease.

Aplastic Anemia or Aplastic Crisis—Decreased red blood cell count due to the bone marrow factory temporarily shutting down. The most common cause is a virus called Parvovirus B19.

Bilirubin—A yellow-orange chemical produced from the breakdown of hemoglobin, when red blood cells break down.

Bone Marrow—Inside of your big bones, the marrow has cells that can make red blood cells, white blood cells, and platelets.

Bone Marrow Transplant—A procedure that kills the existing bone marrow production and plants donor (usually a matched brother or sister) marrow by transfusion. The bone marrow begins to make blood cells according to the genetic code of the donor. This has cured over 600 sickle cell patients.

Carrier—One who inherits only one gene for a genetic problem like sickle cell. Usually there are no symptoms, and the carrier will never have the disease. Two carriers of sickle trait have a 25% risk of having a child with sickle cell disease.

Chromosome—The DNA code for all the parts of the human body. Each person has 46 individual chromosomes in cells, 23 donated from each parent. Chromosome 11 is where the sickle cell mutation occurs.

Complete Blood Count (CBC)—A blood test that gives information about how many red cells, white cells, and platelets a person has in their bloodstream.

Cord Blood—This is the blood remaining in the umbilical cord and placenta after a baby is born and the cord is cut. This blood is rich in stem cells that can be saved and used in transplants.

Folic Acid or Folate—A B vitamin necessary for making new red blood cells. It also acts as a vasodilator, which allows your blood to flow more freely through small blood vessels, and it helps homocysteine level, which may reduce your risk of complications, such as stroke, leg ulcers, and heart attack. Most sickle cell patients should take 1 mg a day. It is found in green, leafy vegetables, fruits, and whole grains.

Gallbladder—A pouch in the right upper abdomen under the liver. It stores bile to help digest fats in the diet. The gallbladder can be removed if it is full of gallstones and causing problems.

Gallstones—Too much bilirubin from red blood cell breakdown can cause stones to form in the gallbladder. This can cause pain in the right upper abdomen, nausea, and indigestion when eating fatty foods.

Genes—These are the basic units of inheritance. They are located on chromosomes.

Gene Therapy—Treatment that will change the genetic defect or the gene product (hemoglobin) in sickle cell disease. The first experimental studies of gene therapy for human sickle cell disease started in 2014.

GVHD (Graft-versus-host disease)—GVHD can occur after a bone marrow or stem cell transplant when someone receives bone marrow tissue or cells from a donor and the donor's immune cells attack some of your organs. Before a transplant, tissue and cells from possible donors are checked to see how closely they match the person having the transplant. The closer the match, the less likely GVHD is to occur. Treatments to help prevent GVHD may include immunosuppressants, antibiotics and sometimes steroids. Symptoms of GVHD normally occur within 12 months of the transplant and can include skin rash, nausea, diarrhea, jaundice, dry eyes, dry mouth, weight loss and many others.

Hemoglobin—The protein substance inside the red blood cells that holds and releases oxygen. This is where the sickle mutation occurs.

Hemoglobin AS—This is sickle cell trait. The inheritance of one normal hemoglobin gene and one sickle hemoglobin gene.

Hemoglobin Electrophoresis—The blood test that identifies the type of hemoglobins present in the red blood cells.

Hemoglobin S Beta Thalassemia—This is a type of sickle cell disease in which one inherits an S gene and a beta thalassemia gene from his or her parents. S beta0 thalassemia is more severe than S beta+ thalassemia.

Hemoglobin SC—A type of sickle cell disease in which one inherits an S gene and a C gene from the parents. This causes sickle cell complications, with increased eye and bone problems. Life expectancy is longer than with hemoglobin SS.

Hemoglobin SS—This is called sickle cell anemia and is the most common form of sickle cell disease.

Hemolysis—The breaking apart of red blood cells. Normal red cells last 120 days; sickled red blood cells last about fourteen days.

Hydroxyurea—The first medication for sickle cell disease that increases fetal hemoglobin. It reduces pain events by one half, the need for hospital admissions, absences from school or work, the need for blood transfusions—and it prolongs the lifespan.

Intravenous (IV)—A small plastic catheter placed in a vein to allow water, blood, or medication to enter the blood stream directly.

Jaundice—A yellow color in the white part (sclera) of the eye produced by increased bilirubin in the blood. Usually caused by increased red blood cell breakdown in sickle cell patients.

Magnetic Resonance Imaging (MRI)—Taking pictures of the brain or other organs of the body with a large magnet-based device.

Pain Episode or "Crisis"—Pain in the bones and muscles where blood flow has been blocked by sickled red blood cells.

Port-a-cath (also other brands like InfusaPort)—An under-the-skin port that requires only a one-time needle stick that allows long-term painless access to sample venous blood, and/or to give IV fluids and medications.

Prenatal testing—ways to check a pregnant woman to determine if the baby has sickle cell disease or another genetic problem. Here are 2 common ways: Chorionic Villus Sampling (CVS) is done when the pregnancy is 10–12 weeks along. A catheter or needle is used to get a sample of the placenta for testing. Amniocentesis is done when the pregnancy is 15–18 weeks along. A sample of fluid is drawn from the womb.

Priapism—A prolonged painful erection of the penis from trapped sickled red blood cells.

Pulmonary Hypertension—The condition in which the lungs' blood vessels are abnormally tight and raise the blood pressure there.

Reticulocyte Count or Retics—The count of brand new red blood cells just released from the bone marrow factory. It is the best indicator of how the bone marrow factory is producing red cells.

Retina—The back of the eye, where light is detected. The blood vessels of the retina can be weakened or blocked by sickle red blood cells. A retina exam with (eyedrops to dilate the pupils) should be done every year for teens and adults. This can lead to bleeding in the eyeball, and loss of vision.

Sequestration—Blocked blood flow from sickled red blood cells in the spleen or liver. Blood can flow in, but it cannot flow out. This causes weakness, abdominal pain, and swelling of the liver or spleen.

Spleen—An organ in the left upper area of the stomach that helps filter germs from the blood stream.

Stroke—Blocked blood flow to an area of the brain that can cause weakness, numbness, trouble speaking, or trouble thinking. Stroke is a medical emergency.

Transcranial Doppler (TCD)—a special ultrasound device that uses painless sound waves to check for blocked blood flow in the brain. "Transcranial" means that the ultrasound wavs go through the skull to capture This test can identify children at greatest risk of having a stroke.